MENOPAUSE

HOW TO GET YOUR LIFE BACK AND RID THOSE NEGATIVE SYMPTOMS ONCE AND FOR ALL

ROSE MARIE ACOSTA

Menopause: How to Get Your Life Back and Rid Those Negative Symptoms Once and For All

Copyright © 2019 by Rose Marie Acosta

Disclaimer:

CONTENTS

ABOUT THIS BOOK

My name is Rose Marie Acosta and I have been a health enthusiast for over 30 years (I'm 54) and now a certified keto health coach. This book is about my journey going through menopause and the peri-menopause side of it as well. I discuss my lifestyle and the challenges I went through as I tried to find an answer to my suffering both physically and emotionally. I also share my eating journey and how I discovered keto as a sustainable way of eating and how it brought healing to my body from the menopausal symptoms I suffered with. Last, but not least I share how I healed emotionally by changing bad habits and finding new ones that brought positivity in my life.

From the night sweats to the hot flashes along with many other symptoms, I discuss how you can begin to heal your body with the simple methods I used.

Sure, we are all different and what works for me might not work for you but isn't it worth a try?

You are valuable, and your life depends upon your wellness both physically and mentally. My goal is to teach as many women as I can what I have learned and how to get relief through diet, nutrition, wellness, and exercise.

I myself suffered alone and I know some of you do too. I recall doing research looking for the cure to my ailments, only to discover that peri-menopause and menopause symptoms can last anywhere from 4-18 years combined. Talk about misery!

Can you imagine what it would feel like to get rid of that fatigue you have been feeling for years? How would it feel to be more energetic and play with your grandchildren? Or, maybe for you, it is just enjoying a nice walk or going up and down stairs with less pain. What about losing that last stubborn 10-20 pounds? I'm sure at least one of these symptoms you can relate to.

Whichever one it may be, I will show you how to apply my system to your life, so you will get the best possible results from the symptoms of menopause. Will you join me?

PREFACE

MY PERSONAL
HEALTH JOURNEY

I love health and wellness. It feels great to feel great. It wasn't always this way for me. I wouldn't say I suffered from poor health because I always found solutions for what ailed me. I popped a lot of ibuprofen for pain and drank lots of coffee to stay awake.

My pain happened gradually and over time caught up with me.

It all started here…

One day at work as a daycare provider, I reached down to pick up a small piece of something on the floor, and I soon realized I couldn't get back up-I was literally stuck in a bent-over position.

I remember hearing, "What's wrong, Ms. Rose?" from the voice of one of the toddlers in my care. As I slowly made it to the floor I said, "Ms. Rose just needs to sit down." I was in excruciating pain.

Eventually, I went to a doctor because my back hurt so much, and I also had developed a limp. I was diagnosed with sciatica. I went through three months of physical therapy, and I think I was the biggest grouch during those three months of recovery.

I soon realized my body could not remain in a youthful state forever, and if I wanted to remain youthful, I had to act. I thought to myself, *I can't let this happen again*, so I started exercising.

Exercise became my best friend. Any chance I had (keep in mind I was a stay-at-home mom raising my own children in addition to running a home daycare) I would exercise. Whenever the kids napped, I would be in the living room doing aerobics. I would watch Denise Austin-she was in great shape and that's what I wanted.

This was fine at first but because I didn't wear shoes while exercising (*what was I thinking?*), I eventually tore some ligaments in my right knee. After one year of not being able to walk without experiencing significant pain, I decided to have the surgery that was initially recommended.

Luckily, I didn't have to have a knee replacement. Instead, I underwent laparoscopic surgery in which the doctors were able to laser out the tears that occurred. The therapy I received after surgery brought some relief but my knee never quite healed. It stayed in a swollen state that lasted for years. I learned to live with one knee fatter than the other–I always had fat knees, oh well. ☺

As time went on, I continued working out but always had to ice my knee right after. Getting older brought more aches and pains. Refusing to live like this I continued to search for answers.

I've always been a-health enthusiast-eating well, sleeping, and taking my vitamins but I always ended back at the drawing board. I longed for the feelings of youthfulness, the days of feeling alive and energetic. *What happened?*

I was determined to find the solution no matter the cost. I tried all the following: Jenny Craig; Atkins diet, Weight Watchers, low fat/nonfat, count calories, etc. At first, they worked but I would always go back to my old way of eating. I worked out five days a week–still no weight loss.

I was trying so hard to no avail. Pushing forward, I knew I couldn't give up. I read about mineral deficiencies causing symptoms in people and recalled hearing about how American soil is depleted and there aren't many nutrients in it. I ran across a documentary once with an elderly doctor explaining how people could avoid stroke, Alzheimer's, obesity, and diabetes because they were all caused due to a lack of certain minerals.

At the time, it made sense to me, but it was unclear what I should take and how much. That part stumped me. As my journey continued, I came across another way of eating called Paleo. It interested me because

I heard so many great things about it. I decided to try it.

After one year on the Paleo diet, even though strict, I still found myself craving sweets and salty things. I eventually "fell off the wagon" and cheated from time to time (which I didn't like at all). I only wanted to feel satiated after my meals and not have food on my brain all day. I occasionally would stumble across "ketogenic eating". I thought it was considered a caveman way of eating and that it would be impossible to pull off.

There was a series that was advertised in my email called, "The Real Skinny on Fat." It was 20-plus hours of interviews with doctors and people in the health field who were discussing their knowledge of the keto diet. I watched all the episodes and was blown away. I soon discovered that keto was a way of life, not just a diet plan to lose weight.

Sure, you can lose weight while being on keto, but it also brings healing to the whole body just by changing what you eat. I became brave one day and jumped in full force. I listened to YouTube videos and read a lot about it. The first two weeks I came down with the keto flu, but I was persistent. I started noticing amazing changes–swelling in my right knee gone, brain fog–gone, craving sweets and salty foods–gone. I also noticed I wasn't so irritable or achy either.

After so many years of searching, I finally found my answer. I soon started to share my experience with friends and family. One day on Facebook, I noticed there were health coach certification courses being offered. I didn't know that a health coach was a profession, and I became even more excited. I wanted so much to be a health coach, so I could spread the word about this new healthy way of living.

Before jumping in I asked some of my adult children what they thought. It was unanimous, they all confirmed it would suit me and felt I had always been a health enthusiast in some shape or form. Immediately after that confirmation, I looked into a couple of programs and signed up for one.

After many months of studying, I am now pleased to say I am a fully certified keto health coach and I love it. I have learned so many wonderful things about the human body and how it works. Things make sense now. I long to share this valuable information with other women so they can also experience relief from some of the terrible symptoms of menopause.

I no longer take ibuprofen for pain or drink coffee just to stay awake. I continue to eat healthy, exercise, and enjoy my life now. Do I still have days where I experience menopausal symptoms? Yes, I do occasionally, but not nearly as before. So, yes, I can confidently say I love health and wellness and it does feel great.

CHAPTER 1

EATING IS THE KEY

What should I eat?

Oh, how I love to eat. I think I spent the majority of my life with food on my brain. I never realized the impact every bite and drink has on the body. I guess in youth, everyone thinks they are invincible. Well, I was definitely that person.

A definition of Food: *"That which is eaten to sustain life, provide energy and promote the growth and repair of tissues; nourishment."* -Eric Berg, DC

Think about that definition for a moment. What we eat should sustain life, provide energy, and promote the growth and repair of tissues; it is our nourishment. Our society is addicted to eating fast food because we live in a fast-paced world, and we have developed a microwave mentality-Do we really believe that the fast food we-eat nourishes our body? How about the soda we consume? I wonder what vitamins are in that? What about energy from the food we eat?

Maybe we get a little energy from the coffee we drink or the sugary carbs we consume. But how long does that last? Maybe an hour or two? Lastly, what about growth and repair of tissues? I don't think the growth part is talking about our obesity. What food could possibly repair our tissue? What I am about to share with you is what I believe to be a lifestyle of healthy eating that can bring about energy, sustainability, nutrition, and the promotion of growth and repair of tissues. Before I share what, I eat, I would first like to share the remarkable results I have had by changing my eating habits. They are:

1) Inflammation/Aches/Pains in Different Parts of the Body:

I had reoccurring inflammation around my right knee after a surgery I had about 14 years ago. After two weeks on keto, it completely went away. Other aches and pains such as joint pain also went away.

2.) Tiredness/Fatigue

I was always tired no matter how much I slept. I was especially tired right after a meal and would need caffeine to keep me up. Fatigue was ceaseless. Now, I have plenty of energy and no longer need naps to keep me up.

3) Always Hungry/-Never Satisfied Even If Full

No matter what I ate, I always had a feeling of never being satisfied. I eat two-three times a day now and feel fully satiated from one meal to the next.

4) Salty/Sweet Cravings

This was a daily occurrence. I no longer have these cravings.

5) Brain Fog

At times, I felt like I was on another planet. I lacked mental clarity, my focus was off-, and I suffered from irritating-forgetfulness, even with small things like number sequences, -zip codes, and-badge numbers-at work. I now have clarity in my thinking and the cloud has been lifted.

6) Weight Gain-Cannot Lose Weight

After my second pregnancy, I easily gained ten pounds for each child I had and it seemed impossible to lose (keep in mind I have six kids). I have lost 26 pounds and have kept it off.

7) Hot Flashes/Moodiness

Hello peri-menopause and menopause. I've had hot flashes for over 10 years, and in the last couple of years, it had gotten really bad. Each day I felt extreme moodiness and experienced between 30-50 hot flashes. Now, I can sometimes go a full day without one-and they are very mild. My irritability and moodiness went away too.

8) Heart Palpitations

I suffered from this for years (maybe over 20 years-from-nutritional deficiency). Now, I rarely get a heart palpitation, and if I do, it always has something to do with my food intake. Maybe I hadn't eaten enough vegetables the days before or didn't get the sleep I needed.

9) Anxiety/Depression

I also suffered from this for over 20 years – (Also due to nutritional deficiency). This was my toughest battle out of all my symptoms. It was tough because right when I thought it was gone it would come back. Kind of hard to explain, it would creep up on me without notice. I would suddenly feel very sad and a feeling of hopelessness would come over me. I thought, - *"if only I could think more positive thoughts I could win this battle."* However, it was not just my thought life I needed to change but lifestyle changes as well such as sleeping, eating, and exercise. After incorporating keto eating and these new lifestyle changes, I now have a sense of wellbeing that doesn't go away. I truly believe anxiety and depression are a thing of the past and a battle conquered.

The first couple of weeks transitioning to a low-carb, healthy ketogenic way of eating was all by trial and error. I didn't know what I was doing but knew I wanted to be healthy. I jumped in quick and immediately cut out all refined carbs and even fruit. I didn't have much energy as a result, but eventually, my body adapted.

If you decide to take the plunge

It takes time to transition the body from burning sugar as fuel to burning fat for fuel, so try and not be so hard on yourself during this time. I don't recommend jumping in as I did. I think taking things slow the first week or two will work better. For example, instead of cutting out all refined carbs the first week, cut out half of them. Instead of eating 6-8 times per day, eat only three times and add a little fat to each meal like real butter or olive oil. Taking baby steps will ensure an easier transition for you. As time goes on, you can become a little stricter with your carbs. The next week, cut your sugars in half again until you no longer desire them. Eventually, you will not have a taste for them. If you do, continue to increase your fat intake. This will rid your cravings.

Once you are ready, cut out all refined carbs. That includes: rice, pasta, bread, cookies, cakes, doughnuts, etc. You might think, Wait a minute! I love sweets and breads, but here's the good thing-you can continue eating these foods. More on that later.

Eat 7-8 Cups of Veggies Per Day

I know this sounds like a lot, and it is, but your body needs the nutrients and minerals from vegetables, especially potassium. The recommended dietary allowance (RDA) of potassium is 4,700 mg. a day. To give you an idea, one banana has 300 mg. of potassium. That's a lot of bananas if we want to meet the daily requirement.

Cruciferous veggies like broccoli, cauliflower, and Brussel sprouts are probably the best choices because they contain phytonutrients and potassium. Phytonutrients act as extra protection for our cells to fight off disease. If you are not able to eat these particular vegetables, -experiment with what best suits you.

At first, I started at about 3-4 cups per day. This was even a challenge since I rarely ate veggies, some lettuce and tomatoes here and there or a big salad maybe once a week. I now can confidently say I eat about 7-8 cups of vegetables a day. What I typically eat in a day is a five-cup salad for lunch and a 2-3-cup spinach smoothie with my dinner. You can eat vegetables raw, sautéed, (in real butter), baked, or steamed. There are many varieties and recipes to try.

A little tip I learned about spinach: On average, 1 cup of raw spinach leaves contains 167 milligrams of potassium, while 1 cup of cooked spinach contains 840 milligrams. Six cups of -cooked spinach- is 5,040 mg. of potassium. Just eating that will give you a little more than your daily recommended requirement.

Have an Adequate Amount of Protein

Eat 3-6 oz. of protein per meal. Excess protein can spike insulin (I will discuss insulin and insulin resistance in the next chapter). Pre-keto, my main food aside from carbs was protein-and lots of it. I currently stay away from barbequed meats as the sauce has a lot of sugars. I love eggs. There are so many ways to prepare them: scrambled, over-easy, poached, omelets, and boiled. I eat 2-3 eggs per meal on most days.

Another favorite of mine is bacon. I enjoy that from time to time with eggs. I will eat about 3-6 slices of bacon. It's a good fat for your body and helps to keep you full throughout the day. I also enjoy a hamburger or cheeseburger, especially when dining out. Instead of having it with bread, I ask for it to be lettuce wrapped. I also enjoy "wild-caught" salmon or canned sardines, both rich in Omega 3.

Keep Your Insulin Low

To keep insulin levels low and lose weight, you must keep your carb consumption below 50 grams per day. Most people think it cannot be done, but that is far from true. When consuming 7-8 cups of veggies per day, I go by the net carbs, which means you subtract the grams of fiber from the total grams of carbs to get your net count.

-For example:

4 cups of spinach (or lettuce of your choice) = approx. 2.5 net carbs

1 cup of broccoli = approx. 5 net carbs

1 cup of tomatoes = 9 net carbs

1 cup of bell pepper = 7 net carbs

Total cups = 7 cups @ 23.5 net carbs

On Sweets and Bread

This was one of my main concerns before diving into keto. I thoroughly enjoyed cookies, chocolate, bread, pasta, and rice. I learned right away there are great substitutes, and I could eat them without guilt.

You can Google keto recipes, try them out and soon you will find the ones you enjoy the most. My favorite bread is Ezekiel bread. It is low carb and gluten free, made from baby sprouts. I don't eat it every day, but I will make a sandwich here and there using it.

To replace rice, I use grated cauliflower. For pasta, I make zucchini spirals or spaghetti squash. I eat it with spaghetti sauce or lightly sautéed in -grass-fed- butter. I still experiment with various cookie recipes. I no longer have those sugary cravings, but the habit is still there, it's nice to have a cookie, cake, or pie recipe on hand for those days I want to indulge. I suggest you add them to the end of your meal-you know dinner with dessert.

A sweet spot for me is 30-50 grams of fat per meal, but you will need to experiment to figure out what's best for you. For example, if you notice you are hungry in between your first and second meal, increase with more fat the second meal. Continue this with each meal until you are no longer hungry in between. I started out eating three meals per day, and now I am totally satisfied with eating twice per day, which is lunch and dinner. The body has a chance to rest when you do this. It also brings healing to the body.

Types of fat that are good for you:

Grass-fed butter;

Extra-virgin-olive oil;

Grass-fed cheese;

Avocado/Avocado oil;

Nuts-walnuts, pecans, etc.

I have shared with you the different ways of eating healthier, so it is up to you to make the right choices. With consistency and a positive mindset, you will get better at it. You will also find that you are no longer interested in the things you once ate.

CHAPTER 2

WHY IS SUGAR SO BAD?

Insulin and Insulin Resistance

Sugar is the culprit behind many diseases. It comes in sweet little packages in all different shapes and sizes, but it wreaks havoc on our body. Every time we consume sugary carbs, it raises our insulin levels. Insulin is a hormone created by the pancreas to regulate sugar in the blood.

"The average American consumes 26-31 teaspoons of sugar a day." – Eric Berg, D.C.

That is a lot of sugar!

Insulin will carry sugar into our cells for fuel, and any excess will store as fat. Overtime, if we continue eating a high carb diet we may experience the following symptoms:

Brain fog;

Irritability/moodiness;

Sugar and salt cravings;

Need naps after meals;

Fatigue and lack of energy,

And, if sugar consumption is not controlled, will eventually lead to a condition called insulin resistance. This is when the receptors on certain cells in our body are resistant to receiving insulin. This means increased glucose in the blood, which produces even more insulin. Higher levels of insulin present in the blood signal energy to be stored in fat cells, resulting in weight gain. The following conditions can also occur:

Obesity;

Diabetes;

Heart Conditions;

Stroke;

Fatty Liver;

Cancer;

Alzheimer's,

I have good news.

If we change our eating habits as mentioned in my previous chapter, we may reverse much of the damage that has been done. As a result, we may begin to experience the following:

Clarity in thinking;

Better mood;

Weight loss;

More energy;

Cravings stop;

No need for naps after meals;

Inflammation goes away.

Now after hearing that, which would you prefer?

One of the primary purposes of fat is to prevent the body against the starvation of sugar. When carbohydrates are not available for fuel your body will use fat as a backup energy source. As long as we keep insulin levels low (and stress), we will continue to burn fat as fuel.

Keep healthy snacks available like cookies and cakes, made with natural sweeteners and almond or coconut flour. When you get tempted to eat a sugary treat, you can quickly eat what you've already made and feel fully satisfied without guilt. This is a great way to keep insulin levels low as well.

CHAPTER 3

SLEEP

Sleeping has got to be one of the best things to do besides eating. Most of my life, I never had a problem with sleeping. I would lay my head on a pillow and within literal seconds, fall asleep.

About ten years ago, I started getting night sweats. I would wake up in the middle of the night, and my whole body would be drenched in sweat, my clothes soaked. I would toss the blankets off only to find myself freezing from all the dampness. This lasted for years.

As this tapered off, I noticed that I would wake up every night between 1 and 3 a.m., and my mind would race with all these different thoughts. I would use the bathroom and attempt to go back to sleep, but after tossing and turning, I soon realized I could not go back to sleep and would get up and get ready for work instead.

Occasionally, I would go back to sleep for maybe 15-20 minutes before my alarm clock would go off. On those days, I was exhausted at work and-irritated. I even felt angry at times-angry because I was so tired from the night before.

I remember drinking lots of coffee throughout the day just to stay awake. That didn't help, but my body was desperate for energy. In addition to the coffee, I would crave sweets and salty foods. Lack of sleep causes an increase in appetite (especially to eat carbs), which adds on the extra pounds.

I soon started getting hot flashes too. Those were just as bad as getting night sweats except instead of getting soaked, it would feel like my whole body was on fire, -especially my face. It was embarrassing because I would get a hot flash in the middle of a conversation with someone.

I remember once when I felt a hot flash coming on, I quickly excused myself and made up some excuse to avoid being seen with a bright red face. These were all signs of menopause, and I hated it. I tried a couple of over-the-counter remedies, but they never really helped me.

I shared my frustration with a co-worker friend of mine about not being able to sleep, and she suggested I take magnesium. She gave me some of hers, maybe ten days' worth. I started taking them right away. That first night, I recall having the best night of sleep I had had in years. The magnesium even helped with the heart palpations I had been having for quite some time. They seemed to lessen with taking this supplement.

As I shared earlier, the night sweats eventually stopped, but I continued having hot flashes, and they would keep me up at night. I started taking 5HTP on some nights and that would help some, but I still struggled to get a good night's sleep.

When I finally changed over to keto-and started using relaxation techniques along with exercise, I began to sleep soundly throughout the night. Now the times I do wake up, I can easily go back to sleep.

Our Body Needs 7-9 Hours of Sleep Daily

Sleep is like nutrition for the brain. Most people need between 7 and 9 hours each night. I'm sure you have heard of REM sleep. There is also delta sleep. Delta waves occur in the brain during the 3rd and 4th stages of sleep causing delta sleep, which is a deep sleep. Women experience delta sleep more than men, but it declines with age. Research has found that women have more delta waves than men. Another interesting fact is the Ketogenic diet can cause delta wave increases which means a deeper sleep. Our body burns fat during our deep sleep so if we are not deeply sleeping we are not burning fat.

Naps are also good to take, -especially power naps. No more than 30 minutes is considered a power nap. If you sleep longer than that, you will feel groggy. Healing takes place when we sleep. Our heart rate drops and our blood pressure lowers.

When we get a good night's sleep, we are also rejuvenated the next day and have more energy for the tasks that lie ahead. Sleep also aids in the prevention of accidents due to fatigue.

Ways to Get Restful Sleep

Along with eating a healthy keto diet, take supplements to aid with sleep if you need to. Magnesium is great to take about one-hour before going to sleep. As we age, our serotonin levels decline, so taking 5HTP or L-tryptophan (same family) triggers the body to produce serotonin, therefore resulting in a better night's sleep. You can find these supplements at most health food stores. Eventually, you will find what works best for your body and in no time, you will be on the road to a great night's sleep.

CHAPTER 4
EXERCISE

Exercise can be a love-hate relationship. Either you love it or hate it or a little bit of both. Just as eating is a lifestyle, so is exercising. I only became a fan of exercising after getting a bout of sciatica. My physical therapist told me I would be more susceptible to it unless I stayed in shape to prevent it from happening again.

There are two types of exercise, aerobic and anaerobic. I'm not talking about the aerobics from the eighties where you have on the leg warmers and onesie with a headband. The one I'm talking about includes, -walking, yoga, jogging, and Pilates. You can hold a conversation while doing this type of exercise.

The other type, anaerobic,-means without air, like sprints or high-intensity interval training. It means it is difficult to talk while doing these exercises. Both burn sugar and fat. Sugar will immediately be burned, and then fat burning will take place 14-48 hours after exercise during deep sleep.

Like I mentioned in the previous chapter, make sure to tackle your sleep right away with supplements and relaxation techniques. This will aid in feeling better throughout the day. I walk five days a week (20-25 minutes at work and on weekends) and do a variety of exercises such as Pilates, HIIT, or Yoga 2-3 times per week. I also do a lot of stretching.

Depending on where you are at physically, you can start out slow and gradually build it up over time. You can start out by taking short walks then gradually over time increase the length and intensity like walking up hills and stairs. This will increase your muscle tone. It's easy on the body and enjoyable. Walking also promotes better sleep because you are moving every part of your body, and this keeps circulation going to clear the mind.

CHAPTER 5

SUPPLEMENTS

Growing up, I always believed that vitamins were for old people. Keep in mind, this was through the eyes of an adolescent. I started taking them when I became pregnant with my first child. It was a prescription for pre-natal vitamins given to me by my gynecologist. Once my baby was born, I stopped taking them.

Over the years, I took a multivitamin daily. That didn't last because I never knew exactly what it did for me. I didn't notice a change, so I figured, *What's the use?*

When peri-menopause hit -in my forties I started experiencing night sweats. I believed this something I had to experience because of aging. I investigated a number of remedies, such as some over-the-counter products and various vitamins, but they didn't bring relief. There are so many vitamins in the market and it's hard to know which ones to take. You must be careful though, because 90% of all vitamins are synthetic:

> *Man cannot duplicate what nature creates, even when the chemical analysis is identical. Most vitamin supplements are isolated chemical USP (United States Pharmacopeia) vitamins and minerals pressed together in a pill. The vitamins are produced synthetically from petroleum in chemical plants, while the minerals come from mining companies.*
>
> *Synthetic minerals are derived from rocks such as limestone, coral, oyster shell, sand, and chalk. Yum. Although these materials have mineral profiles, our bodies do not absorb them properly. Humans are not designed to digest rocks and oyster shells. Ideally, we should get all our minerals from plants.*
>
> *–Myers, "90% of Vitamins are Synthetic".*

What about the 10%?

The other 10% are whole-food concentrated vitamins/supplements. They come from real food sources. For example, wheat-grass is a good source of vitamins, including vitamin C, vitamin E, iron, calcium, magnesium, and amino acids. You can go to most any health food store and find it in powder form. Another example is nutritional yeast. It contains many of the B vitamins. You can also find this in powder form.

I do not claim to be an expert in choosing the 10% out there, but you can set up some guidelines to steer you in a more positive direction.

1) Read the labels. If the ingredients listed are a short paragraph, chances are it is not good for you.

Study the source of the manufacturer. Do your research. Of course, this is entirely up to you, but you will be amazed at what you find.

2) Get most of your vitamins and minerals from real foods. Choose high-quality foods from grass-fed and organic sources whenever possible. Sure, they might have some pesticides but not nearly as much and as dangerous as most foods out there.

The supplements I use have given me great results, especially magnesium-with taurate. I take two right before bed. I used to take electrolyte powder with potassium when I first transitioned my eating because I didn't eat many veggies. Now that has changed, and I find it no longer necessary.

Over time you'll find your body adapts to your intake of nutrients and reserves them for future use. Experiment with the ones that work best for you where you are at physically in your journey.

CHAPTER 6
POSITIVE THINKING

I have not always been a positive person. In fact, I would say I was a bitter, negative person.

A runaway at the age of 14 only added to my negativity. I truly believed at the time I had to lie and steal my way through life and not trust anyone. I was a high school dropout and addicted to drugs. I'm happy to say that is all behind me now; however, it left a lot of scars. I have since healed from those scars, and I have learned some valuable life lessons.

I didn't like myself. I didn't like how I looked, how I felt, or who I was. Because of this, I'm sure I generated a lot of negativity towards those I was around. I would have a smile on my face, but inside I didn't like anyone. I found my joy in my children-they were my whole world. I knew they loved me, and they depended on me. That was a great feeling.

After surviving two bad marriages, I came to the conclusion that I needed help. I needed help to change my outlook on life. My faith had always gotten me through tough times, but I also knew I had to do something as well.

I have always been a fan of self-help books. Some of my favorites have come from Joyce Meyer. She has gone through great struggles in her life, so I believed she knew what she was talking about and thought her books could help me. I soon learned to believe the best of myself and others no matter what the situation and not to say negative things about myself.

This is easier said than done. But over time, this became a habit of mine. I also went through a time of forgiveness. All the people who hurt me were affecting me because I had so much bitterness against them. I made a list of those people, and no matter how much I didn't want to forgive them, I did.

I would speak it out loud every time they came to mind until it no longer bothered me. This process took years, and as I forgave people, some others would come to mind. People that were buried so deep in my mind that I had forgotten them. I also had to ask some people to forgive me as well.

As my children got older, I noticed I was slowly healing inside. I started to like myself. I recall daily reciting positive affirmations. I still do that to this day. It was a battle at the beginning, fighting off all those negative thoughts that bombarded my mind, but now all those years of working on myself have really paid off. I believe all the positive things I say about myself. This is not in a prideful way but in a healthy way.

Once my mind frame changed about myself, I was able to generate good thoughts and feelings to and about others. Have you ever noticed when you smile at someone their automatic reaction is to smile right back? In the same way, our thoughts have the same effect.

Those bitter, negative days are far behind me now. When a negative thought creeps up, I immediately counteract it with something positive. I believe if you are determined and put in the work to become more positive, it will become a reality in your life. Life's too short, right?

CHAPTER 7

CREATE NEW HABITS AND GET RID OF BAD ONES

Creating new habits and getting rid of bad ones can be a challenge. The first step is identifying those bad habits-then making a conscious effort to change them.

I had a bad habit of being alone. I say it was a habit because I love alone time, and I utilized it often. If I don't spend time with others on purpose, I might get stuck in alone mode. I work at this because I realize we need others.

Create the habit of cultivating new friendships

Women, in my opinion, especially need each other. We love to talk. If you go to a kindergarten playground, you will notice boys running around making plenty of noises. They are engaging in make-believe sword fights or battles, while little girls are talking amongst themselves. You might find some talking out loud, and no one is even there. We just have to talk!

When my children were small, I belonged to a church group, and I always worked in the children's ministry. I did this because my kids would not sit still in the service. I also enjoyed working there because I could talk to other moms. I found we had so much in common during those times.

I always felt good afterward, especially if I was able to connect to someone and chit-chat away while we took care of the little ones. Volunteering is a good opportunity to meet other women with similar interests. I recall once while volunteering at a food pantry, that it wasn't a good fit for me. I wanted it to be, but I only stood around while the director did all the work. I kept asking her what I could I do, but she said: "Don't worry,"- There will be plenty of work to do."-I stayed for four hours and ended up with a sore back after all the standing around. I even tried to talk with the other volunteers, but it was only small talk and never amounted to much.

That volunteer position was not for me. Ladies, it's okay to try something even if it's not a good fit. Eventually, you will find something you truly enjoy. Unless you get out there and try, you will never know. Your next best friend could be at that volunteer event.

I also volunteered at the church giveaways during Christmas and Thanksgiving. We would give food and presents away to those in need, and it was enjoyable to see these families so happy.

Exercise classes are also a good place to meet friends. It might take a few times of going to the same class but so worth it.

Find and hang out with women who are positive and support you. There's nothing worse than hanging out with someone negative or who complains all the time.

Sometimes, at work, you might encounter negative people. I had a job before that seemed like I was at a high school. The amount of gossip that was going on was terrible. I learned to stay away from certain people. Eventually, I became friends with positive people and ended that negative cycle. Be careful who you surround yourself with because they can be damaging to your health. Toxic people are everywhere, and there is no shortage of them.

You might even have some in your own family. These people tend not to value anyone, and they take and take and will suck the life right out of you if you let them. Instead of leaving them feeling refreshed, you leave feeling like you just ran a 10k marathon, totally drained.

I've had a few of those type of relationships, and they can be the hardest to break for some reason. I seemed to have gravitated toward them when I was at the lowest points in my life. I didn't value myself, so it was easy to allow others not to value me either.

I'm so glad I was able to recognize that and get myself out of those toxic relationships.

Over time, as I improved in my thoughts of who I was, I was able to attract other positive, supportive people.

Staying up late:

Another bad habit that can be damaging to our health is staying up late. I spoke about the importance of getting 7-9 hours of sleep in a previous chapter.

I had the bad habit of staying up until 11 p.m. every night because I would watch a movie, the late news, or a talk show. The next day I would pay the price at work. I did this for years. I now go to bed just about every night at 9 p.m.

We need our sleep. -I call it beauty sleep. The next day after a full night's sleep we will feel a lot more beautiful compared to only getting a few hours. The things we sacrifice to finish a movie. I'm sure you get my point on the importance of sleep.

Whatever your negative habit may be, make a conscious effort to change it to a good one to live a more fulfilled and healthy life. Your body will thank you for it.

CHAPTER 8

MAKE TIME FOR YOURSELF AND OTHERS

Making time for yourself is an important part of self-care, to extend the best version of yourself to others. There are simple things you can do, such as taking a hot bath with Epsom salts. Epsom salts are soothing to the body because they contain magnesium. Treat yourself to a manicure or pedicure. If it is not in the budget, you can do it yourself as well. I do my own nails and toe-nails and on occasion go to a salon. I watched YouTube videos, so I could learn how to do it correctly. It may sound funny, but there is a certain way to file your nails and a certain way to polish them to make them look like you just stepped out of a salon.

With a little practice, you will in no time create a salon-perfected look. Get your hair done or style and trim your own hair. I have cut my own hair before. I watched a few YouTube videos and was able to pull it off but eventually went back to my hairdresser to get my hair evened up, he-he. Getting massages are also a great thing to do. It helps to relieve stress from the body and clears the mind.

My mother has been getting monthly massages for years and swears by them. If you are busy with children and running a home full time, take 10-15-minute breaks throughout the day and relax or meditate. Use this time to reflect on your goals for the day. Maybe do some deep-breathing techniques to let go of stressful situations or events that took place. Remember, we are a work in progress. Enjoy the journey. I often stop throughout my day and give thanks for my family, my job, etc. It keeps me on track not to take this life for granted but to express gratitude. It also puts me in a better mood.

Another thing that brightens my day is flowers. Why wait for someone to buy them for you? There are a lot of stores that sell beautiful bouquets relatively inexpensive.

What I've shared with you are some small ideas of how to bring a little joy to your life and maybe put a smile on your face. You will discover as you apply some of these techniques you will start to feel better about yourself and will soon express those feelings toward others.

Giving is a wonderful expression to share. There are so many ways to give. I'm sure you're familiar with the saying, "It is better to give than to receive." When you give, the return is so rewarding. I belonged to a youth church group many years ago, and we were all challenged to pay someone's way for a meal or movie or any other creative way we could come up with. I decided to pay for the person behind me at the toll bridge. I recall feeling so good about it right after. I did that a few different times, and it was so enjoyable. Even complimenting someone can make someone's day.

Giving comes in all shapes and sizes. Have you heard of the five love languages? Everyone receives love in different ways. One of the love languages is acts of service. That is one of my favorites. I feel so loved when someone does an act of service for me. When my kids were growing up and they would clean the house or take out the garbage without me telling them to, I felt so loved. One of my daughter's love language is quality time so when a friend or family member spends time with her, she feels loved. One of my boys' love language is receiving gifts. If you give him something, he feels loved. We are all wired differently, so make it a goal to find out what the love language is of the people in your life. Try it out and see if it works. Simply asking them what makes them feel loved will also work if they are open and honest. The quiz is still available online, just Google: "The Five Love Language Quiz" and you will be able to take the test.

Share your gifts and talents with others. It may be tutoring children or visiting the elderly. Give the gift of listening. People love to be genuinely listened to. Have you ever engaged in a conversation with someone, and you could tell they really weren't interested in listening to you? It is such an uncomfortable and awkward feeling. Doesn't it feel great when someone really pays attention to you and they listen? Using someone's name in a conversation makes others feel good too. There's something about it when we hear our name being spoken. Avoid giving unsolicited advice. I'm guilty of that one. Maybe it's the mom in me, but I am working on getting better at not doing it as much. Unless someone asks you for advice, don't give it.

Support those around you. I have an elderly neighbor whom I occasionally see in the summertime. Once after I finished doing yard work, I noticed she was trying to trim her rose bush. Weeds had grown all around it, and I noticed the difficulty she had attending to it. I went in my garage and took out my clippers and started helping her trim it. Once the job was finished and I cleaned everything up, she asked me to stay there. She went in her house and brought back a gift of appreciation. It was bag full of dish towels that she had embroidered herself. I thought to myself, *What a beautiful gift*. The time and energy that was put into making them. It was priceless.

There are many charities you can give to as well. I support some children through Children International. I give monthly and support children of third-world countries. The small amount I give provides medical and dental care plus educational resources and support to their families, like providing clothes or pots and pans for cooking. My reward is receiving letters from my sponsored children. It brings a smile to my face or tears of joy when I read their letters of appreciation.

Last, but not least is to spend time on purpose with your family and friends. Family is so important to me. When my kids were growing up, I would spend one-on-one time with each one, so they would know I valued my time with them. A whole hour to do whatever they wanted, without distractions, and I gave them my full attention. We didn't have much money then, so it was a big deal for them to go to Burger King and get a whopper and fries and go to the park and just hang out. Now, my children are grown up and have families of their own, and we still have get-togethers whether it is for birthdays or dinners. This is precious time we share and value.

I'm looking forward to the future outings we will have-and now I get to involve my grandkids too.

Do today what you want for your future. If you want to feel good and remain healthy when you get older, take care of yourself today. Invest in your friends and family today so you can reap the benefits later. Remember to always be generous and your rewards will find you.

I want to thank all who read this book as the proceeds will go to a worthy cause. I have a heart for children that are sexually exploited and trafficked. That's why I am donating 100% of the proceeds from this book to Project GRL. It is a program through Joyce Meyer Ministries. One of their goals is to fund and support initiatives that rescue, educate and restore women and girls impacted by this insidious evil. This is a tragedy in our world today, and I want to give whatever I can to help save and rescue these precious children. Plus, the strategies in this book can be life-changing for those who apply them to their lives. I wish you all the health and wellness this life has to offer.

WORKS CITED

Berg DC, Eric. The New Body Type Guide: Get Healthy, Lose Weight & Feel Great.

Bracy, Kate, and Np. "How Long Will Menopause Last for You?" Verywell Health, www.verywellhealth.com/how-long-will-menopause-last-2322698.

"Does Sleep Affect Weight Loss? How It Works." WebMD, WebMD, www.webmd.com/diet/sleep-and-weight-loss#1.

"Menopause." Womenshealth.gov, 18 Mar. 2019, www.womenshealth.gov/menopause/.

Myers FDN-P, Wendy. "90% of Vitamins are Synthetic." Myers Detox, https://meyersdetox.com.

Wickham, Erica. "How Much Potassium Is in Raw Spinach?" LIVESTRONG.COM, Leaf Group, www.livestrong.com/article/530709-how-much-potassium-is-in-raw-spinach/.